Michelle P.

MW00512404

Gluten - Free Vegetables Recipes

50 Quick And Tasty Recipes For Gluten-Free Vegetables For The Whole Family

© Copyright 2021 by **Michelle Parker**

WARNING

The information in this book is for informational purposes only. It is not medical advice or medical opinion and should not be construed as such in any way. Before starting the Sirt diet or taking the foods and/or supplements recommended for this diet, always seek advice from a trusted physician or qualified nutritionist. This is essential to avoid possible side effects. We disclaim any responsibility for any ailments or problems should you decide to follow the Sirt diet or take any foods or supplements associated with this diet.

Table of Contents

Michelle Parker

Michelle Parker

Gluten Intolerance

Definition

Gluten intolerance is a Para physiological condition of altered intestinal tolerance to a protein nutrient, called gluten.

The term "celiac disease" or "c(o)eliac" comes from the greek "koiliakos κοιλιακός", which means "abdominal"; this term was introduced in 1800 to translate an ancient Greek description of the so-called disease of "Areteo of Cappadocia".

Gluten intolerance is NOT an allergy, neither to gluten, nor to other wheat proteins or the like.

While it is true that it involves the intervention of the immune system (like allergies), it is also true that celiac disease does so in a totally different way than allergic forms. Gluten intolerance causes a localized complication in the mucosa of the intestine and, only later, leaves some traces on the blood type parameters. However, even in the most important cases, the involvement of allergy-specific antibodies (IgE) is missing and there is no risk of anaphylaxis.

More than a disease, gluten intolerance is preferably defined as a Para physiological condition, since, in the absence of exposure to the specific agent (gluten), the organism remains quietly in homeostasis as if it were healthy. Otherwise, a pathological picture of extremely variable severity and symptoms may arise.

Difference between celiac disease and gluten intolerance

Those who suffer from celiac disease have a very specific type of injury to the intestine, in which the complex proteins of wheat, rye and barley induce the immune system to attack the small intestine, while those who suffer from gluten sensitivity does not have this type of injury, but still feel the inflammation caused by gluten.

The difference between the two disorders is therefore given by the different immune reaction to gluten. In gluten sensitivity, the body's main immune defense (innate immunity) reacts to the ingestion of gluten by fighting it directly, i.e. causing inflammation in the digestive system and other parts of the body. In celiac disease gluten is, instead, fought by both innate and adaptive immunity, that is, by the most sophisticated part of the immune system. Communication problems between the cells of the adaptive immune system cause these cells to fight the tissues of the body, resulting in the atrophy of the intestinal villi associated with celiac disease.

What to eat in case of gluten intolerance

Unfortunately there is no cure for gluten intolerance, but it is possible to live with this condition by following a specific diet, avoiding to consume foods containing this substance. Gluten is found in: wheat, spelt, barley, rye, oats and in all products derived from them such as: bread, pasta, crackers, breadsticks, cookies, cakes, breadcrumbs, yeast, barley coffee and substitutes, malt, beer, soy sauce, cutlets, broth preparations, frying preparations, ice cream preparations and in some cold cuts.

Here is a list of foods that can be consumed by individuals with gluten intolerance:

amaranth, buckwheat, legumes (beans, lentils, peas), corn, millet, quinoa, rice/wheat rice, sesame, soybeans, tapioca, potatoes, chestnuts, all meats, all fish and shellfish, ham, aged cheeses, eggs, vegetables, fruit, butter, lard, extra virgin olive oil, olive oil, peanut oil, soybean oil, corn oil, sunflower oil, grape seed oil, walnut oil, salt and herbs, dried and fresh mushrooms, olives, milk (not mixed with other ingredients), fresh cream, low-fat whole or fruit yoghurt without added cereals or malt, brewer's yeast, roasted ground coffee, tea, chamomile, carbonated soft drinks, nectar and fruit juices, wine, sparkling wine, champagne, grappa, tequila, cognac, brandy, Scotch whisky, cherry, Jamaican rum, port, marsala, sugar, honey.

To be avoided are: Wheat (wheat), spelt, bulgur, oats, kamut, barley, spelt, rye, triticale, sorghum, cous cous, malt and cereal flakes where malt has been added, floured and breaded foods, frozen products (except whole uncleaned fish) if contaminated in processing, surimi, floured nuts, coffee substitutes containing barley, balsamic vinegar, apple cider vinegar, beer, non-Scottish whiskey, vodka, gin and spirits such as bitters, infusions, curry, seitan, cereal and malt yogurt, and soy sauce. For a complete and official list of gluten-free foods suitable for celiac and intolerant people we recommend consulting the AIC handbook: a publication published annually that collects, after evaluation, even products that, although not designed specifically for a particular diet, are still suitable for consumption by celiac.

Gluten Free Vegetables

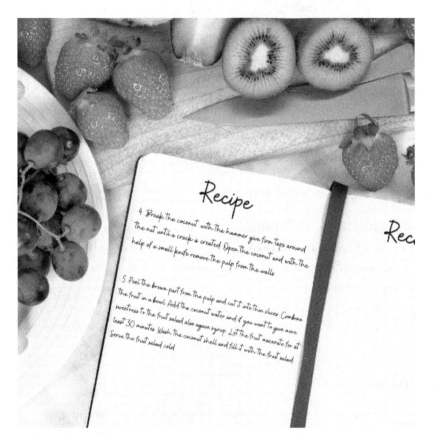

Vegetable Meatloaf

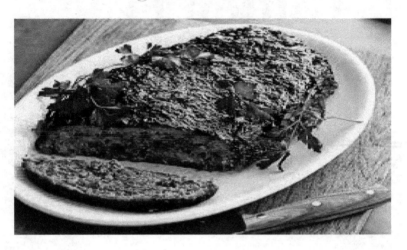

Ingredients for 6 persons:

- 500 grams of Potatoes
- 250 grams of Ricotta
- 5 teaspoons of Parmesan cheese
- 3 Courgettes
- 3 Carrots
- Salt

Preparation

1. To prepare the vegetable meatloaf, take the potatoes and, after washing them, boil them for 20 minutes in lightly salted water. Then cut the carrots and zucchini into cubes and cook them for 20 minutes in a steamer.
2. Once cooked, remove the skin from the potatoes and mash them with a potato masher. Then add the vegetables, ricotta cheese and salt to the bowl.

3. After mixing all the ingredients well, add the Parmesan cheese and, with the help of parchment paper, form the meatloaf. Bake it in a plumcake mold for about 30 minutes in a hot oven at 180 degrees.

4. After letting it cool a bit 'here is ready to enjoy your delicious vegetable meatloaf.

Potato Parmigiana

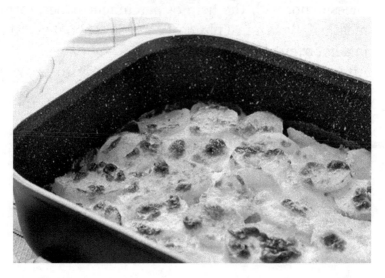

Ingredients for 6 people

- 250 grams of Ragout
- 200 grams of Mozzarella
- 1 kilo of potatoes
- Extra virgin olive oil
- Oregano
- Salt

Preparation

1. In order to prepare the potato parmigiana as first thing you must boil potatoes in boiling water for about 20 minutes. Once the time has passed, remove the skin, let them cool for a few minutes and cut them into slices. Then prepare the Bolognese sauce.

2. Pour a few tablespoons of sauce into an oven-proof dish, make the first layer with the potatoes and add salt, then slice the mozzarella.

3. Place the mozzarella on top of the potatoes and continue alternating layers of meat sauce, potatoes, a pinch of salt and mozzarella. On the last layer of potatoes pour extra virgin olive oil and sprinkle salt and oregano.

Sweet and sour onions

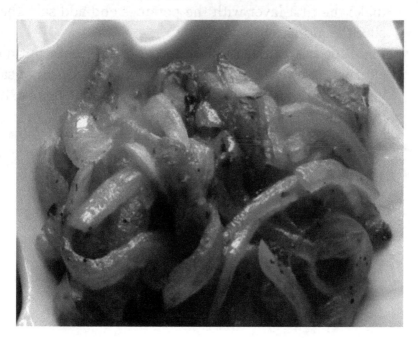

Ingredients for 4 people

- 250 onions
- 60 millilitres of water
- 50 milliliters of balsamic vinegar
- 3 tablespoons of caster sugar

Preparation

1. To prepare the sweet and sour onions put 2 tablespoons of sugar in a pan, add water and melt over low heat.
2. Take the onions, wash them under water, add them to the pan and cook 5 minutes covered with a lid.
3. Add the balsamic vinegar, stir and add another tablespoon of sugar. Cook for 10 minutes without lid.

4. When the cooking time is up, let them cool and then your sweet and sour onions are ready to be enjoyed.

Chard parmigiana

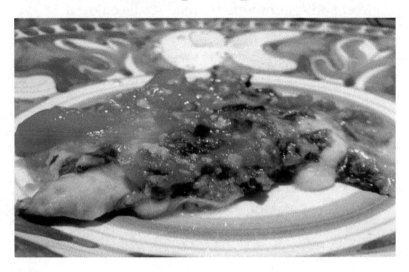

Ingredients for 4 people

- 500 grams of chard
- 1 package of tomato puree
- 2 tablespoons of extra virgin olive oil
- 2 nuts of butter
- 4 fillets of anchovies
- 2 cloves of garlic
- parsley
- 16 slices of gouda cheese
- salt and pepper

Preparation

1. Clean the chard by removing the ribs. Cut the latter into rounds and wash them together with the whole leaves under running water in order to eliminate any residual soil.

2. Blanch the leaves in plenty of salted water. It will only take a few seconds: when the leaf turns bright green, it is time to remove it from the water and place it on a plate wide open so that it does not stick. Proceed in this way with all the leaves

3. In the same water in which you blanched the chard, boil the ribs. 10 minutes will be enough. Drain the chard and melt the butter in a non-stick pan with the garlic and anchovies.

4. Add the boiled chard ribs and sauté for a few minutes. Add the tomato puree and season with salt and pepper. Flavor with chopped parsley and cook for about ten minutes. Meanwhile, turn on the oven at 170 degrees.

5. Now compose the dish: brush with extra virgin olive oil and lay the first chard. Sprinkle it with the tomato and then with a slice of cheese cut in half, covering it with another chard leaf. Complete each oven dish with 4/5 layers until you finish the leaves. Place a few curls of butter on top and bake for 25 minutes.

Spicy Carrots

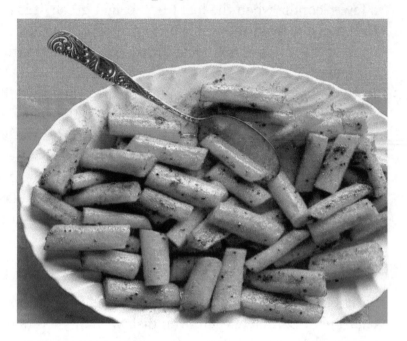

Ingredients for 4 people

- 700 grams of carrots
- 2 cloves of garlic
- 2 spoons of extra virgin olive oil
- 1 hot chili pepper
- 100 millilitres of Armagnac
- 100 millilitres of water
- 2 anchovies
- butter
- chopped parsley
- pepper
- salt

Preparation

1. Clean the carrots by removing the skin and ends then cut them into rounds as similar in size as possible. Peel the two cloves of garlic and chop the chili pepper.
2. Heat the oil in a frying pan and add the garlic and chili pepper. Add the anchovy fillets and, with the help of a wooden spoon, let them melt until they disappear.
3. Add the carrots and stir to season. Now add the Armagnac, stir and allow the alcohol to evaporate for a couple of minutes so that the scent of the liqueur remains.
4. After the alcohol has evaporated, close with a lid and let it cook for 10 minutes. When the time is up, add the water and continue cooking for another 10 minutes with the lid off. Remove the garlic cloves
5. Add the chopped parsley and stir. Stir in a couple of knobs of butter to make the sauce creamy. Serve piping hot.

Marinated cherry tomatoes

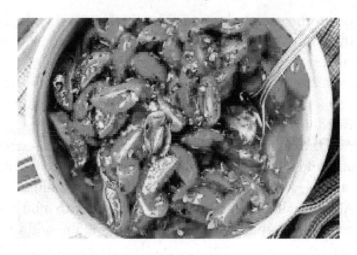

Ingredients for 4 people

- 1 kilo of cherry tomatoes
- 1 handful of fresh rosemary
- 1 handful of fresh basil
- 2 cloves of garlic
- extra virgin olive oil
- salt

Preparation

1. To prepare the marinated cherry tomatoes, wash the cherry tomatoes and dry them, then cut each in half and place them in a bowl. After that, proceed with the seasoning and marinating. Season the tomatoes with half of the fresh rosemary needles, a clove of garlic cut into small pieces and a sprinkling of salt, without exaggerating.
2. Add a drizzle of extra-virgin olive oil and stir, then let them rest for about 20 minutes, so that they take all the flavors.

Once the marinating time has elapsed, drain them from the liquid they have lost and place them on a baking sheet covered with parchment paper. Place the tomatoes with the skin in contact with the baking sheet and the seeds facing upwards. Bake in a preheated oven at 180 degrees for at least 70 minutes.

3. After the cooking time, turn off the oven and let them cool inside, then remove them from the pan and place them in a bowl where you are going to season them again with fresh herbs. Start by breaking up the basil and fresh rosemary with your hands.

4. Continue by adding the second clove of garlic and finally season them again with a generous amount of extra virgin olive oil and finally mix them well and let them rest at least one night before adding them to your dishes.

Pan-fried peppers

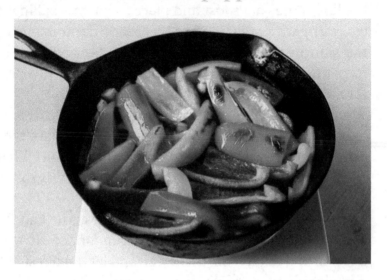

Ingredients for 4 people

- 5 Peppers
- 1 onion
- 100 millilitres of White Wine
- 50 millilitres of Extra Virgin Olive Oil
- Salt

Preparation

1. To prepare the peppers in the pan, take the peppers, I chose yellow, but you can also use red ones, wash them and remove the green stem, the white central part and all the seeds. Then cut them into slices.
2. Take the onion, remove the skin, cut it first in half and then in thin slices.

3. Put the extra virgin olive oil in a frying pan, heat for 2 minutes and add the onion slices. Sauté for 3 to 4 minutes and then add the peppers. Add salt and white wine.
4. After cooking 30 minutes over high heat, the peppers are ready in the pan.

Eggs in purgatory

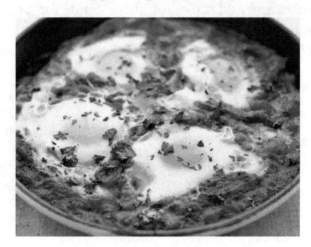

Ingredients for 1 person

- 1 egg
- 300 grams of peeled tomatoes
- 3 basil leaves
- 1 pinch of chilli pepper
- 2 cloves of garlic
- extra virgin olive oil
- 1 pinch of salt
- pepper

Preparation

1. Place a frying pan over low heat in which you will pour the extra virgin olive oil and then the cleaned and grated garlic. Add to the garlic a pinch of chilli pepper and fry over a very low flame without letting anything burn.
2. Pour the peeled tomatoes into the lightly browned mixture and, as soon as they come to the boil, mash them with a

fork in order to obtain a smooth sauce in small pieces. Let the sauce simmer for about ten minutes over low heat, then add the basil, washed and roughly chopped, and add salt. Let it cook for about five more minutes without allowing the tomato to dry out too much.

3. Once the sauce is cooked, it will be time to add the egg as well, so remove the pan from the heat and crack the egg into the pan (if you are making more than one, place them far apart from each other), then place the pan back on the heat and turn up the heat, cover with a lid and let go just long enough for the egg white to thicken, leaving the yolk soft and creamy. As soon as the egg is ready, remove from the heat. Add a pinch of salt and a generous grinding of pepper, and serve the dish while still hot.

Imam Bayildi

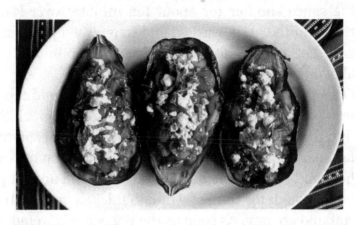

Ingredients for 4 people

- 4 eggplants
- 300 grams of cherry tomatoes
- 3 teaspoons of tomato paste
- 1 medium onion
- thyme
- salt
- 2 cloves of garlic
- chopped parsley
- water
- 2 handfuls of pitted black olives
- 2 handfuls of pitted green olives
- 4 anchovy fillets
- 2 tablespoons of extra virgin olive oil

Preparation

1. Start by finely chopping the onion. Then divide the green and black olives into coarse pieces and crush the garlic

with the garlic press. Alternatively, chop it very finely with a knife.

2. Cut the cherry tomatoes into four wedges. If they are already small, divide them in two. Heat the oil on the stove and fry the anchovy fillets until they melt. In the meantime, cut the eggplant into thick slices.

3. When the anchovies have melted, add the chopped onion and garlic and brown them. Add the chopped parsley and olives. Cook for a few minutes to flavor the oil well.

4. Add the tomato paste and let it dissolve then add the cherry tomatoes. Add a splash of water to mix all the flavors together and cook the tomatoes slightly. Close the lid and continue cooking for 10 minutes.

5. Turn on the oven to 180 degrees so that it reaches temperature. In the meantime, heat a cast iron skillet with a pinch of salt and thyme. Grill the eggplant slices on both sides, then place them on a drip pan and spoon the sauce over each slice. Bake for 15 minutes. Before serving, sprinkle with parsley and a drizzle of oil.

Omelette with cooked ham and stracchino cheese

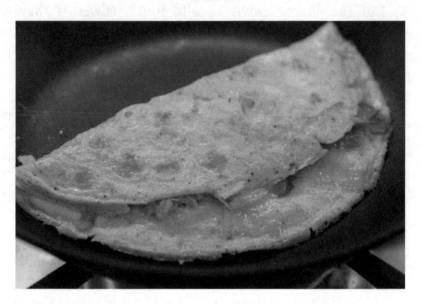

Ingredients for 2 people

- 4 Eggs
- 4 slices of cooked ham
- 100 grams of Stracchino
- 1 handful of Parsley
- Salt
- 30 grams of grated Parmesan cheese
- Extra virgin olive oil

Preparation

1. In a bowl, beat the eggs. Finely chop the parsley and add it to the beaten eggs. Then incorporate the Parmesan cheese.
2. Heat a few tablespoons of oil in a frying pan, keeping the flame at half its capacity. Pour the eggs into the pan

recreating a circle and let it cook for two minutes, then turn it upside down.

Snow peas and potatoes

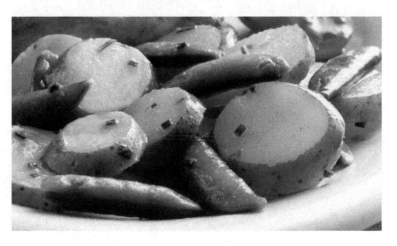

Ingredients for 4 people

- 400 grams of Potatoes
- 600 grams of Snow Peas
- 1 Onion
- 1 clove of Garlic
- 1 Chilli Pepper
- Salt
- Extra Virgin Olive Oil
- Rosemary

Preparation

1. Snow peas, or mange-tout peas, should be eaten tender and with their skins on, just start by removing the ends and washing them well in cold water. Boil them in salted water for about 5 minutes, then drain and set aside.
2. Peel the potatoes and soak them for a few minutes so that the excess starch comes out. Sauté the onion, garlic and

chili pepper in a few tablespoons of oil. As soon as the onion is soft and blond, add the drained potatoes.

3. Season the potatoes with the rosemary, cover and cook over high heat for at least 12 minutes. Remove the lid and season with salt, allowing them to brown well until a crispy crust forms, then add the snow peas and finish cooking over medium heat for about 7 minutes more. Serve your side dish hot.

Sweet and sour peppers

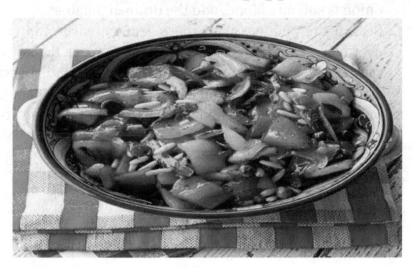

Ingredients for 6 people

- 2 Yellow Peppers
- 2 Red Peppers
- 3 tablespoons of caster sugar
- 1 glass of white wine vinegar
- 4 tablespoons of Extra Virgin Olive Oil
- 5 Anchovy fillets
- Salt and Pepper

Preparation

1. Take the peppers, wash them carefully and dry them. With a knife cut them in half, clean the inside of the peppers trying to eliminate all the white part and the seeds. Cut them into slices at least a couple of centimetres wide, then proceed to divide them into three pieces in a rather coarse manner.

2. In a high-sided pan, put the olive oil and sugar and caramelize over low heat until the sugar has completely dissolved and is quite dark in color. Add the chopped peppers and let them cook for about 10 minutes, stirring gently from time to time.

3. Add the wine vinegar and let it cook for another 10 minutes. Separately, prepare the anchovy fillets to complete the dish. Remove from the heat and leave to cool in a casserole dish. Serve warm with a few anchovy fillets as decoration.

Eggplant pizzaiola

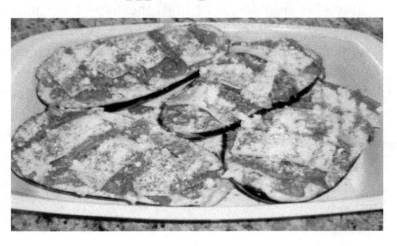

Ingredients for 4 people

- 4 Aubergines
- 600 grams of Tomatoes
- 4 cloves of Garlic
- 8 leaves of Basil
- 200 grams of Pasta Filata cheese
- 30 grams of grated Parmesan cheese
- 2 tablespoons of Extra Virgin Olive Oil
- Salt
- Seed oil

Preparation

1. First prepare the sauce, then crush the garlic cloves and remove the skin, brown them in extra virgin olive oil and add the washed and diced tomatoes with all their skins. Cook for about fifteen minutes and when cooked, add a little salt and set aside.

36

2. Peel the eggplants and cut them in two lengthwise first and then each half into three parts. Heat enough seed oil in a frying pan and cook the eggplant, salting lightly on all sides. Once they are golden brown, drain them and let the excess oil drip off.

3. Place the eggplant in an ovenproof dish and cover with the tomato sauce, then garnish with the washed basil leaves. Bake at 220°C for at least 18 minutes.

4. Once the cooking time has elapsed in the oven, remove from the oven and sprinkle the surface with stringy cheese and grated Parmesan on top. Bake again for 2 minutes and remove from the oven.

Mulinciani 'mbuttunati (stuffed eggplant)

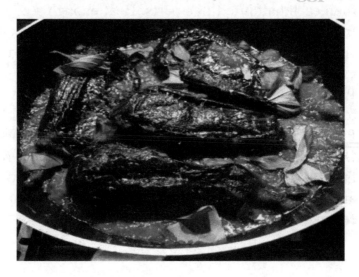

Ingredients for 4 people

- 8 Eggplants
- 16 cloves of garlic
- 300 grams of Caciocavallo Ragusano cheese
- 1 liter of tomato puree
- 50 millilitres of extra virgin olive oil
- 250 millilitres of water
- Salt and Pepper
- Basil

Preparation

1. Start by washing and cleaning the eggplant, then remove the stalks. Prepare all the ingredients for the stuffing, then slice the cheese, wash and dry the basil, clean and thinly slice the garlic cloves and finally mix salt and pepper in a single compound. Take the washed eggplant and make

4

Michelle Parker

four deep vertical cuts on the belly and one in place of the stalk.

2. In each cut, place a little salt and pepper, followed by a few slices of garlic and a piece of cheese.

3. Finally, stuff each eggplant hole with plenty of fresh basil. Heat the oil in a frying pan and brown all the eggplants. Once done, transfer them to a very large pot.

4. In the pan with the leftover oil, bring the tomato puree and 250 ml of water to a boil, add salt and add everything to the pan along with the eggplant, then transfer to the heat and let it cook, covered and over medium heat, for at least 70 minutes; once this time has elapsed, uncover the pan, lower the heat and let it cook for another 20 minutes, allowing the sauce to reduce. Serve this dish warm, accompanying the eggplant with the cooking sauce.

Cucumber boats with robiola cheese

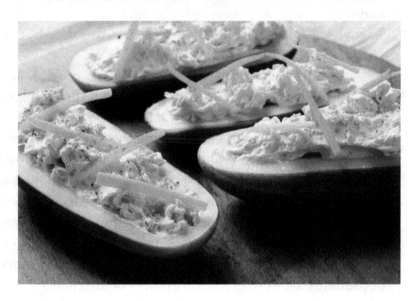

Ingredients for 4 people

- 2 Cucumbers
- 50 grams of Robiola
- 10 grams of Capers
- 1 Tomato
- 1 tablespoon of Extra Virgin Olive Oil

Preparation

1. Fundamental will be to wash and peel the cucumbers, then divide them in half by the long side and remove all the seeds with the help of a digger or a teaspoon.
2. In a bowl, combine the robiola cheese with the finely chopped capers and oil, then knead the cheese until it is well mixed with the capers.

3. Divide the cucumber into portions and fill the part where you removed the seeds with the processed robiola. Wash and cut the tomato in half and remove the seeds, then cut it lengthwise and make strips as if they were sails. Stick the tomato pieces in toothpicks and place them on the boats with the cheese. Serve this appetizer well chilled.

Baked Ratatouille

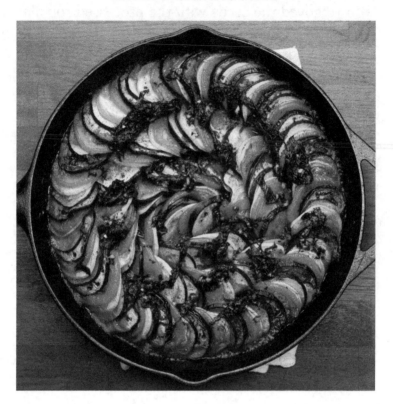

Ingredients for 4 people

- 200 grams of Zucchini
- 400 grams of Eggplants
- 2 Peppers
- 1 Onion
- 1 handful of Thyme
- 2 Tomatoes
- 1 handful of Parsley
- 6 tablespoons of Extra Virgin Olive Oil
- Salt

Preparation

1. Wash and dice the zucchini, then place them in the baking dish. Clean the peppers by removing all filaments, wash them well and cut them first into strips and then into cubes, then place them in the baking dish. Then do the same with the eggplants.
2. Clean the onion and coarsely chop it, add it to the vegetables. Add the diced tomato, chopped parsley and thyme.
3. Season with salt and add the oil, then mix well and bake in a preheated static oven at 250°C for 15 minutes and then at 180°C for the remaining 15 minutes. Serve the ratatouille still hot.

Mushroom eggplants

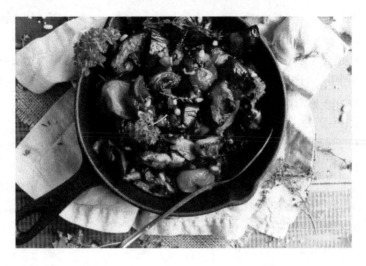

Ingredients for 4 people

- 2 Aubergines
- 3 Tomatoes
- 2 Cloves of Garlic
- 1 teaspoon of Extra Virgin Olive Oil
- 500 millilitres of seed oil
- 1 handful of Basil
- 3 teaspoons of Salt

Preparation

1. Wash and cut the eggplant into chunks, place them in a colander and sprinkle with salt. Leave them for 30 minutes, then squeeze them with your hands to remove the excess water they have released.
2. Cut the tomatoes into cubes. Wash the basil leaves and leave them in cold water for 10 minutes. Pour the oil into a

44

frying pan (the amount of oil should be enough to cover the eggplants).

3. Fry the eggplant a few at a time in hot oil. When they begin to brown, remove them and place them on a baking sheet to drain off the excess oil. Throw away the oil used for frying and, also using the same pan, fry the garlic in a drizzle of extra virgin olive oil. Add the tomatoes, stir and cook for about 3 minutes.

4. Add the eggplant, lower the heat, cover with a lid and cook for five minutes over low heat. Dry the basil and add it to the eggplant. Stir, turn off the heat and let stand 10 minutes before serving.

Eggplant caponata

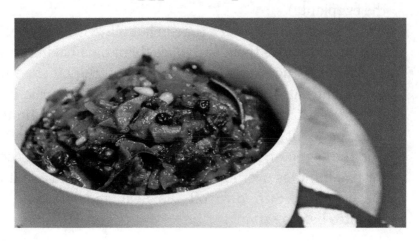

Ingredients for 4 people

- 800 grams of Eggplants
- 300 grams of Tomatoes
- 200 grams of Green Olives
- 30 grams of pine nuts
- 20 grams of Capers
- 300 grams of Red Onion
- 200 millilitres of seed oil
- 2 tablespoons of Sugar
- 60 millilitres of Red Wine Vinegar
- Basil
- Salt
- Extra virgin olive oil

Preparation

1. Wash and clean the eggplants, then cut them first into thick slices and then into cubes. Arrange them in layers in a bowl and salt each layer without exaggerating, then let

them rest for half an hour so that they lose their bitterness. After this time, wash and drain them, then dry them well.

2. Heat the seed oil in a frying pan and when hot, cook the eggplant. Once they are golden brown, drain them and let them lose the excess oil.

3. Clean the onions and cut them into rounds along with the celery, then heat the extra virgin olive oil in a frying pan and brown them. Once they have softened, add the green olives and let them take on flavour for a few minutes.

4. Continue adding the pine nuts, capers and finally the tomatoes that you have washed and diced, then salt.

5. Let the tomatoes cook for about fifteen minutes, then add the eggplant and let it cook for a few minutes. Add sugar and vinegar, let it evaporate and remove from heat. Serve the caponata cold and with plenty of basil.

Grilled zucchini

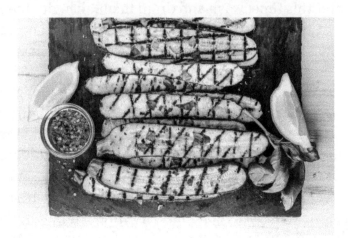

Ingredients for 4 people

- 600 grams of Zucchini
- 250 grams of Red Onion
- 50 milliliters of White Vinegar
- 20 millilitres of extra virgin olive oil
- Mint
- Salt

Preparation

1. Wash and trim the zucchini, then slice them with a thickness of 3 millimetres and if too long divide the slices in half.
2. Heat the griddle and cook the zucchini one minute per side and once cooked, transfer them to an ovenproof dish and season with salt.
3. Heat the oil in a frying pan, slice the onion coarsely and place it in the pan, then season with salt, cover and cook

for about ten minutes, stirring occasionally, until cooked through and soft.

4. Add the vinegar to the onion and simmer over medium heat for 5 minutes, then turn off the heat and add the chopped mint, mix in the sauce and pour over the zucchini. Let them cool and before serving let them sit for at least 12 hours.

Omelette with asparagus and smoked provola cheese

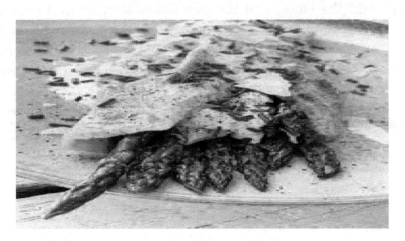

Ingredients for 1 person

- 2 Eggs
- 1 tablespoon of grated Grana Padano cheese
- 3 slices of smoked Provola cheese
- 15 Asparagus
- 1 tablespoon of extra virgin olive oil
- Salt and Pepper

Preparation

1. Break the eggs into a bowl, season with salt and beat them with the prongs of a fork. Add pepper and grated Parmesan cheese and mix with the eggs until smooth.
2. Put the extra-virgin olive oil in a non-stick frying pan and heat it up. When it is hot, but not boiling, pour in the egg mixture. Spread it inside the pan with a spatula and cook for a couple of minutes over low heat. When the edges of

the omelette begin to set, place the three slices of smoked provola over the entire surface.

3. Immediately arrange 11 asparagus on half of the omelette and then fold it in half using a fork and a spatula. Let it cook a couple of minutes more, turn off the heat and transfer the omelette to a plate. Garnish with the remaining asparagus and serve the omelette piping hot.

Lampascioni omelette

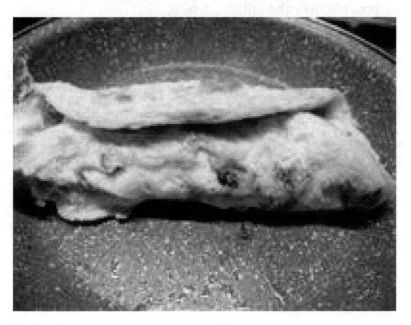

Ingredients for 2 people

- 3 Eggs
- 200 grams of Lampascioni
- 30 grams of grated Pecorino cheese
- 1 tablespoon chopped Parsley
- 2 tablespoons of Extra Virgin Olive Oil
- Salt
- Pink Pepper

Preparation

1. Boil the lampascioni, cleaned and washed, by placing them in a pot with cold water, bringing to a boil and letting them cook for 20 minutes. Put them to drain and let them dry

and cool. Meanwhile, break the eggs into a bowl and season with salt and freshly ground pink pepper.

2. Add the grated pecorino cheese and beat all the ingredients with a fork until the cheese is well incorporated into the eggs. Add the chopped parsley.

3. When the lampascioni have cooled and dried, cut them into wedges and add them to the eggs. Mix well until the mixture is smooth.

4. Pour the extra-virgin olive oil into a non-stick frying pan and let it warm up slightly. Then pour in the lampascioni mixture. Spread it evenly in the pan and level it off.

5. Cover the pan and let it cook slowly over a gentle flame. When the surface of the frittata has almost completely set, slide it onto a plate.

6. With a quick and decisive move put it back into the pan, turning it upside down. Let it cook for a few more minutes and then turn off the heat. Transfer the omelette to a plate and bring it to the table. Cut it into slices in front of the diners and distribute it on the plates.

Asparagus on a bed of potatoes

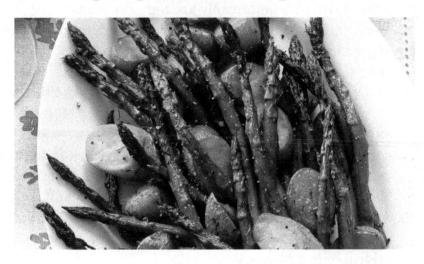

Ingredients for 2 people

- 250 grams of potatoes
- 500 grams of Asparagus
- 1 Lemon
- Salt and Pepper
- Marjoram
- 4 tablespoons of Extra Virgin Olive Oil
- 500 millilitres of water

Preparation

1. Wash the potatoes and place them in a pot. Cover with water, salt and cook for 10 minutes. Wash the asparagus by rubbing them with your fingers under running water. Cut off the bottoms of the asparagus to remove the tough, woody parts.

2. Tie the asparagus into a bunch with a loop of kitchen twine so that they are equal height. Fill the bottom of the pot with water. The water should cover only the stalks of the asparagus, while the tips will steam. If you don't have a tall pot to hold the asparagus "upright" create a tinfoil dome to cover them or lower them slightly by turning the bunch and cover with a lid. Cook over medium heat for about 15 minutes.

3. Grease the baking dish with oil. Drain the potatoes. Cut them into very thin slices without peeling them. Arrange the slices on the baking sheet.

4. Pepper and salt the slices. Sprinkle with marjoram, drizzle with oil and bake in a preheated oven at 200 °C for about 40 minutes. Gently remove the asparagus from the pan, remove the string and place them on the freshly baked potatoes. Sprinkle with lemon and serve hot.

Omelette with potatoes and pecorino cheese

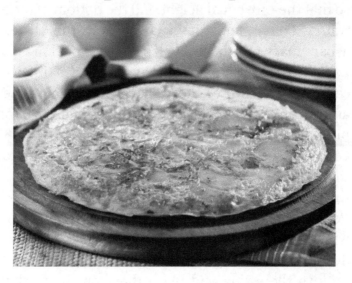

Ingredients for 2 people

- 250 grams of potatoes
- 80 millilitres of Oat Milk
- 2 Eggs
- Salt and Pepper
- 30 grams of Pecorino cheese
- 2 teaspoons of Extra Virgin Olive Oil
- 300 milliliters of water

Preparation

1. Steam the poached potatoes for about 12-15 minutes. Whisk the 2 eggs with the salt and add the milk.
2. Mix milk and eggs well. Grate or chop the pecorino cheese.
3. Peel the potatoes and chop them finely. Heat the oil in a frying pan and arrange the potato slices one on top of the other.

4. Fry the potatoes for a minute. Pour over the eggs and milk and cover with the lid for 5 minutes.

5. When the omelette is puffed up and the top is still moist, sprinkle with pecorino cheese and cover for another minute. Fold the omelette over on itself. Serve the omelette warm with sautéed spinach, bread or a salad.

Roasted mixed vegetables

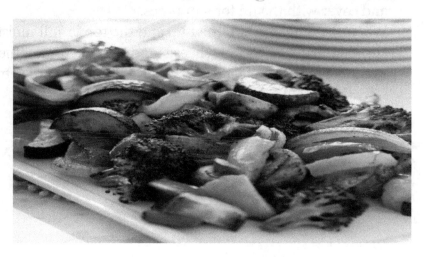

Ingredients for 4 people

- 450 grams of new potatoes
- 2 Courgettes
- 1 onion
- 250 grams of Datterini Tomatoes
- 3 tablespoons of extra virgin olive oil
- Salt
- Rosemary
- Chives

Preparation

1. First proceed with boiling the potatoes, then boil them in salted water for about ten minutes, drain and peel them.
2. Line a baking sheet with baking paper and place the potatoes, zucchini slices and onion on top.
3. Season with salt, add the rosemary and oil and mix the ingredients. Bake at 200 °C in a preheated oven for 35

minutes. At 10 minutes from the end of cooking, add the chopped tomatoes and finish cooking. Just out of the oven add the finely chopped chives to the vegetables.

Vegetable parmigiana

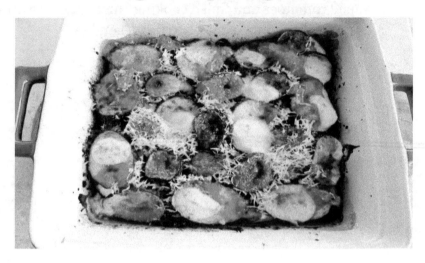

Ingredients for 4 people

- 1 Eggplant
- 2 Courgettes
- 2 Cluster Tomatoes
- 1 Yellow bell pepper
- 1 Red Pepper
- 250 grams of Mozzarella
- 150 grams of Parmesan Cheese
- Salt
- Extra virgin olive oil
- Basil
- Rosemary

Preparation

1. Wash, cut and seed the peppers, place them on a baking sheet with a pinch of salt, a drizzle of oil and some rosemary. Cover them with foil and bake them in the oven

for about 20 minutes at 190 °C. Once cooked, leave them covered for 5-10 minutes, then peel them and cut them into wide strips.

2. Cut the eggplant into discs about 3-4 mm thick, arrange them in a radial pattern and in layers in a colander, alternating layers with coarse salt, place a weight on top and leave them like this for about 20 minutes. After this time, wash off the excess salt and pat them dry with paper towels, then grill them on both sides in a non-stick pan without oil.

3. Cut the tomatoes into cubes and place them in a tall container along with a drizzle of oil and a pinch of salt and blend them with an immersion blender.

4. Cut the zucchini in half and then into thin slices. Cut the mozzarella into cubes and drain off any excess milk. Start composing the parmigiana by spreading some of the raw tomato sauce in an oven dish.

5. Layer the parmigiana alternating the zucchini, cheese, both parmesan and mozzarella, eggplant, peppers and raw tomato sauce until all ingredients are combined. Bake for about 20 minutes at 190°C and serve with a few leaves of fresh basil.

Carpaccio of fennel and pineapple with star anise

Ingredients for 2 people

- 250 grams of Pineapple
- 1 Fennel
- 2 Star Anise
- 1 Lemon
- Extra virgin olive oil

Preparation

1. Place 2 anise stars in a small saucepan and cover with water. Bring to a boil, then lower the heat, cook for about 10 minutes and let cool. Remove the stars from the water: the seeds should come off on their own but the shell should be quite soft. Chop them and let them air dry, then prepare the dressing by combining half of the aniseed reduced to powder, oil and half of the lemon juice. Mix quickly to obtain a frothy and homogeneous sauce.
2. Wash the pineapple under running water. Cut off the two ends and then cut the fruit in half.
3. With a sharp knife, remove the peel, cutting off all the green parts.
4. Slice the pineapple into very thin slices (if you don't have a long, smooth and very sharp knife). Wash and dry the fennel, remove the green tuft and the basal part. Also remove the first layer of the bulb.
5. Cut the fennel in half and slice very thinly.
6. Sprinkle the slices with the other half of the lemon to prevent them from darkening. In a large bowl, combine the

pineapple slices, the fennel, the previously prepared seasoning and the anise cooking water. Leave to macerate for about 30 minutes. Place the slices on a plate, overlapping the pineapple and fennel. Sprinkle with the remaining anise powder and serve.

Pico de gallo sauce

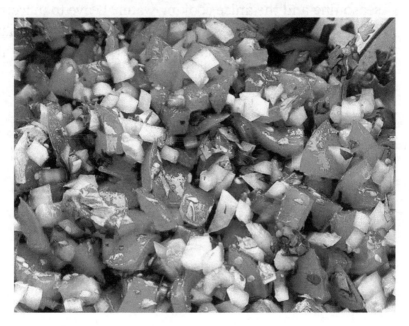

Ingredients for 4 people

- 1 onion
- 3 Tomatoes
- 1 tablespoon of Coriander
- 1 Lime
- 1 Hot Green Chilli
- Salt

Preparation

1. Start by finely chopping the onion and cilantro, after which continue by cutting the tomatoes into small cubes. Place everything in a bowl.

2. Add the lime juice, salt and mix well. Finally, finely chop the hot green chilli and add it to the other ingredients, leaving or removing the inner seeds depending on how spicy you want the sauce to be.

3. Mix everything well but very gently, in order to avoid compromising the final result, which must be a rustic sauce and not blended. Cover the container with plastic wrap and place it in the refrigerator for about 15 minutes, to allow the flavors to blend.

Sweet potato and thyme quenelles

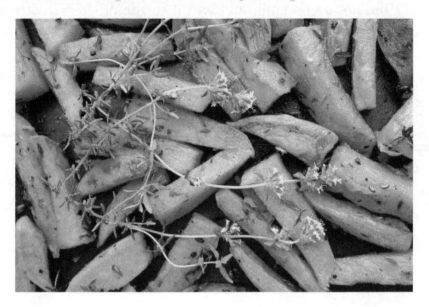

Ingredients for 4 people

- 1 kilo of sweet potatoes
- 20 grams of Maizena
- 1 handful of Thyme
- 1 Egg
- 3 tablespoons of Extra Virgin Olive Oil
- Salt

Preparation

1. Rinse and boil the sweet potatoes in plenty of cold salted water, along with a couple of sprigs of thyme. Once boiled and slightly cooled, peel and chop them, place them in a large bowl and mash them with a potato masher.

2. Add a few thyme leaves, the corn-starch, the oil, salt to taste and mix everything together. Finally add the egg and mix quickly.

3. Now create the quenelles with the help of two spoons of the same size and shape, better if wet, collect some of the dough with one of the two spoons and slide the dough on the other with a rotary movement of the spoons, trying to give the quenelles an elongated shape. Place them on a baking sheet with a drizzle of oil and bake for about 20 minutes at 190°-200°C.

Trifoliated mushrooms with sun-dried tomatoes

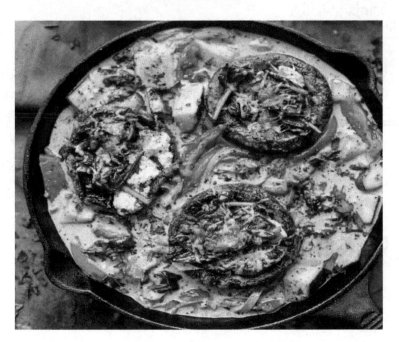

Ingredients for 4 people

- 300 grams of mixed mushrooms
- 8 Dried Tomatoes
- 2 cloves of Garlic
- 1 tablespoon chopped Parsley
- 2 tablespoons of Extra Virgin Olive Oil
- 2 tablespoons lukewarm water
- Salt

Preparation

1. Pour the extra-virgin olive oil into a saucepan. Add the peeled, whole garlic cloves and fry for one minute over

medium-low heat. Add the dried tomatoes in oil, well drained and cut into small pieces.

2. Once you put the sun-dried tomatoes in the saucepan, stir and cook for five minutes, stirring often. Then add the cleaned and chopped mixed mushrooms and let them flavour for a couple of minutes.

3. Sprinkle with salt, add chopped parsley, stir and cook for five minutes.

4. Finally, add warm water and continue cooking for 10 minutes over medium-low heat, stirring often and gently. When cooked, arrange the mushrooms on plates and serve piping hot.

Figs with ham

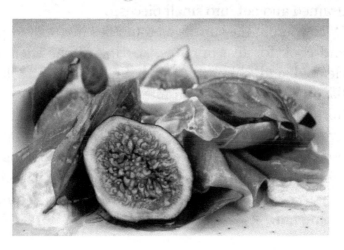

Ingredients for 4 people

- 6 Figs
- 12 slices of ham
- 1 handful of Rosemary
- 1 handful of Rocket

Preparation

1. Wash figs carefully and with great care because they are very delicate fruits, especially when they reach the perfect level of ripeness. Dry them well, again being very careful, with a clean and dry cloth.
2. Divide each fig in half and place it on a serving plate, placing the outer side of the fruit on the plate. Take the ham and wrap a slice around each half, making sure that the two ends of the slice are on the top, then on the inside of the fruit.

3. Secure each slice by wrapping the two ends around themselves and securing with a piece of rosemary sprig. Decorate the plate with scattered arugula leaves and serve immediately.

Salted meat carpaccio with zucchini and Edamer

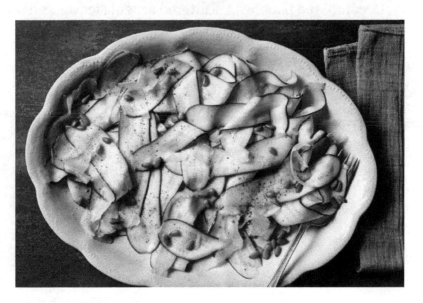

Ingredients for 1 person

- 100 grams of salted meat
- 30 grams of Edamer
- 1 Courgette
- 1 Salt
- 1 tablespoon of Extra Virgin Olive Oil

Preparation

1. Wash the zucchini well and dry it. Remove the two ends and then cut it lengthwise into thin strips and start arranging them on the serving dish.
2. Once you have placed all the zucchini strips, arrange the slices of salted meat on top. Finally place the Edamer slices

on top of the meat: in the center of the plate, one large square slice and the other cut into smaller squares.

3. Sprinkle with salt, drizzle with extra-virgin olive oil and leave to rest for 15 minutes before serving.

Creamed leeks with rosemary

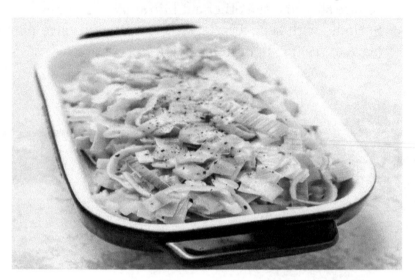

Ingredients for 4 people

- 2 Leeks
- 400 grams of Potatoes
- 1 Onion
- 2 tablespoons of Cream
- 1 handful of Rosemary
- Salt
- Extra Virgin Olive Oil
- Pepper
- Nutmeg

Preparation

1. In a small saucepan, bring 500 ml of water to a boil with two sprigs of rosemary and cook over low heat for 5 minutes to make rosemary water. While the rosemary water simmers, chop the leeks into large pieces and, in a

high-sided saucepan, brown the onion cut into 1 cm chunks with extra-virgin olive oil and a sprig of rosemary.

2. When the onion is golden brown, add the leeks, let them wilt slightly and finally add the diced potatoes.

3. Cook for a few minutes, stirring so that nothing sticks to the bottom, then add the rosemary water with 250 ml of lukewarm water and cook for about 35-40 minutes with a lid and low heat.

4. After the cooking time has elapsed and the water has been reduced by at least half, remove the rosemary and add freshly ground pepper and grated nutmeg directly to the pot. Blend everything with an immersion blender. Once the cream is obtained, mix in the cooking cream and put everything back on the heat for about 10 minutes more, allowing the cream to reduce.

Mexican style beans

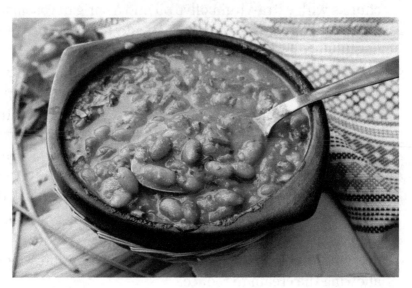

Ingredients for 4 people

- 200 grams of sausage
- 200 grams of Borlotti Beans
- 150 grams of red beans
- 200 milliliters of tomato puree
- 1 onion
- 1 clove of Garlic
- 2 Peppers
- 200 millilitres of Broth
- Extra Virgin Olive Oil
- Salt

Preparation

1. Finely chop the onion and chop the sausage into pieces. Chop the chilies as well, so that you get thin rounds.

2. Pour two tablespoons of oil into a large saucepan and sauté the onion and garlic clove for a couple of minutes, then add the chopped chili peppers and the sausage. Brown the sausage well, stirring constantly to prevent it from burning or sticking to the bottom of the pan.

3. Add the tomato puree and cook for five minutes over medium heat, covering the pot with a lid. Add a ladleful of hot broth and both varieties of beans. Continue cooking for about twenty minutes, adding more broth if the cooking liquid becomes too dry. A few minutes before the end of cooking, add salt to taste.

4. Serve the Mexican style beans piping hot, accompanied by slices of toasted bread seasoned with a drizzle of extra virgin olive oil.

Eggplant and bell pepper rolls

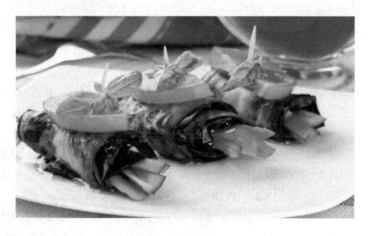

Ingredients for 4 people

- 2 Aubergines
- 2 Peppers
- 2 Tomatoes
- 1 handful of Basil
- Extra Virgin Olive Oil
- Salt

Preparation

1. In a bowl, pour three to four tablespoons of extra virgin olive oil, two pinches of salt and two to three coarsely chopped basil leaves. Mix everything together, cover with plastic wrap and let rest.
2. Thoroughly wash the eggplants, remove the two ends and cut them into slices about an inch thick lengthwise. Cook them on a hot cast iron griddle on both sides.

3. Wash the peppers, remove the stem and cut them in half. Remove the seeds and inner filaments, then cut them into strips.
4. With the help of a brush, preferably a silicone one, grease the eggplant with the basil-flavoured oil previously prepared. Take three to four strips of peppers, place them in the center of each slice of eggplant and roll them up.
5. Wash the tomatoes, cut them in half and then into slices and place one on top of each roulade, securing it with a toothpick. Top with fresh basil leaves.

Eggplant rolls with pine nuts and raisins

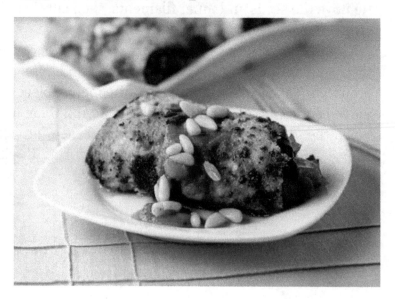

Ingredients for 4 people

- 2 Aubergines
- 200 grams of fresh spreadable cheese
- 2 spoons of raisins
- 2 tablespoons pine nuts
- 1 handful of Chives
- Salt
- Extra virgin olive oil

Preparation

1. Wash the eggplants, remove the two ends and cut them into thin slices lengthwise, then roast them on a cast iron griddle. Alternatively, you can bake them in the oven with a little oil.

2. Put the cream cheese in a bowl and work it in with a fork. Chop the chives and add half of the dose, add a tablespoon of raisins, a tablespoon of pine nuts and, if necessary, a pinch of salt. Mix everything well.

3. Lay the eggplants on a pastry board and spread a teaspoon of the cheese, raisin and pine nut mixture on each. Roll up each eggplant and secure with a toothpick.

4. Place the eggplant on a serving plate and decorate with the remaining pine nuts, the other tablespoon of raisins and the remaining chives. Finish with a drizzle of extra virgin olive oil and serve.

Cucumbers with fresh cheese and cherry tomatoes

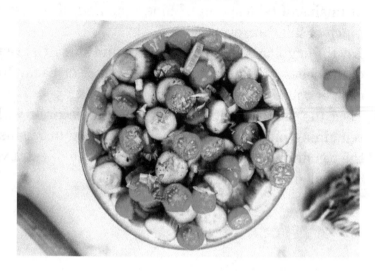

Ingredients for 4 people

- 2 Cucumbers
- 150 grams of fresh spreadable cheese
- 6 Cherry Tomatoes
- 1 handful of Oregano
- Extra virgin olive oil
- Salt

Preparation

1. Cut the cherry tomatoes in half and place them on a baking sheet lined with parchment paper. Pour in a little oil, a generous pinch of salt and bake at 220 °C for about 5-10 minutes.
2. Wash the cucumbers and with the help of a knife or a potato peeler cut the outer skin lengthwise, then leave a

strip of width equal to that of the incision intact and make another. Proceed in this way until you have finished the entire surface of both cucumbers.

3. Remove the two ends of each cucumber and cut them into slices about three to four inches thick. Place them on a serving plate.

4. Place the cream cheese in a small bowl and work it in with a fork. Transfer to a piping bag with a point with a rather large opening and create little tufts of cream cheese on each cucumber slice.

5. Take the cherry tomatoes and place one half on each cucumber. Top with a sprig of fresh oregano.

Mayonnaise

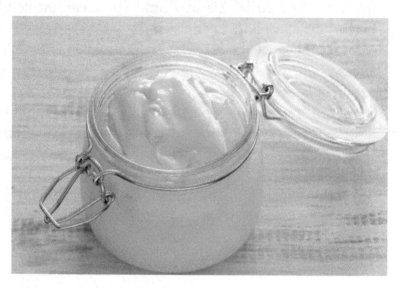

Ingredients for 4 people

- 2 Yolks
- 250 millilitres of Extra Virgin Olive Oil
- 1 Lemon
- Salt and Pepper
- 1 teaspoon of Vinegar

Preparation

1. In a glass bowl place the two egg yolks, add the teaspoon of vinegar, a pinch of salt and, if you like, a pinch of pepper as well.
2. Start mixing with a hand whisk or electric mixer, making sure to always move it in the same direction. Start pouring in the oil drop by drop, or in a trickle, without ever ceasing to mix, taking care not to add too much at a time, otherwise

the mixture will not be homogeneous, or, as they say in the jargon, the mayonnaise will go crazy.

3. Once all the oil has been absorbed, add the juice of half a lemon, a little at a time, and continue to mix, moving the whisk in the same direction. At this point the mayonnaise is ready, adjust the salt and pepper if necessary, pour into a sauce pan and serve, or store in the refrigerator in an airtight container or covered with plastic wrap.

Artichokes with eggs

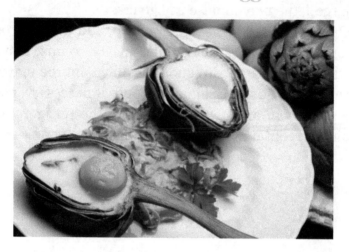

Ingredients for 4 people

- 2 Artichokes
- 5 Eggs
- 1 Lemon
- 50 millilitres of White Wine
- 1 clove of Garlic
- Extra Virgin Olive Oil
- Salt

Preparation

1. Cut each artichoke in half without removing the stem. Wash thoroughly under running water and remove the inner part, i.e. both the part where the classic artichoke hair is usually found and the inner leaves, the more tender ones to be clear. The result must be a sort of bowl in which the egg will be cooked. Throw away the fluff, while the

other edible parts put them in a bowl of water with a few slices of lemon.

2. Rub the inside of the artichokes with half a lemon, put them in a large pot, fill with water and cook for about 10-15 minutes from when the water starts to boil, then drain them, place them on a baking sheet greased with a little oil, spread them slightly with your hands and break an egg inside them. Season with salt and bake at 180 °C for about 10 minutes.

3. In the meantime, cut the inside of the artichokes into julienne strips, brown them in a pan with a tablespoon of oil and a clove of garlic, add the wine and cook for a few minutes, covering with a lid, until tender. Add salt and in a bowl beat well the remaining egg, add it to the mixture and stir continuously until cooked.

4. Remove the artichokes from the oven and place one on each plate, accompanied by a spoonful of the egg mixture and julienned artichokes cooked in the pan. Serve immediately at the table.

Eggplant parmigiana

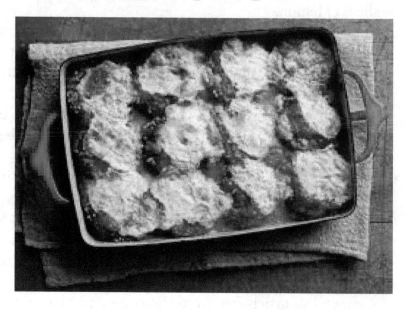

Ingredients for 4 people

- 6 Eggplants
- 300 grams of Mozzarella
- 150 grams of Parmesan cheese
- 700 milliliters of tomato puree
- 1 Onion
- 1 handful of Basil
- Seed Oil
- Extra virgin olive oil
- Salt

Preparation

1. Finely chop the onion and fry it in a pan in which you have poured two tablespoons of extra virgin olive oil. Add the

tomato puree, fresh basil leaves and salt. Cover and cook over low heat for about 20 minutes, stirring occasionally.

2. Wash the eggplants and cut them into slices, not too thin (about one centimetre) lengthwise. Arrange them in layers in a colander, alternating with a teaspoon of coarse salt. Let them rest for about an hour, then wash them well under running water and dry them thoroughly.

3. Fry the eggplants in plenty of seed oil until golden brown. Place them on absorbent kitchen paper.

4. Pour a few tablespoons of tomato sauce into a baking dish and spread it on the bottom. Form a layer of fried eggplant, form a layer of tomato sauce, sprinkle with grated Parmesan cheese and, finally, form a layer with sliced mozzarella. Repeat the operation until all the ingredients have been used up. The last layer should be made up only of tomato and parmesan.

5. Bake at 200°C for about 40 minutes, covering the pan with a sheet of foil for the first 15-20 minutes. Once the parmigiana is cooked, take it out of the oven and let it rest for about 15 minutes before serving.

Purée of potatoes

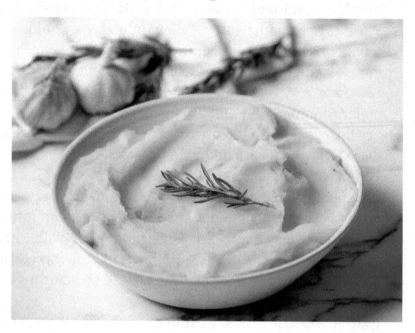

Ingredients for 4 people

- 1 kilo of potatoes
- 400 millilitres of Milk
- 70 grams of Butter
- Nutmeg
- Salt and Pepper

Preparation

1. Wash the potatoes well and place them inside a pot. Fill with water so that the potatoes are completely immersed and boil them until they are completely cooked. To check the cooking you can insert a toothpick or the tip of a knife:

if it sinks completely without effort the potatoes are cooked.

2. Drain the potatoes, peel them while they are still hot, cut them into small pieces and mash them directly into a pan using a potato masher or vegetable mill.

3. Add the chopped butter, nutmeg, salt and pepper and mix well. Heat the milk in a separate saucepan and when it is hot add it little by little to the potato and butter mixture. Add the milk according to the consistency of the potatoes and to your taste, i.e. if you prefer a thicker or thinner mashed potato.

4. Put the pan on the stove and cook over medium-low heat, stirring constantly, until the mashed potato is smooth and homogeneous and until it has reached the desired density. Serve piping hot.

Chunks of potatoes and bacon

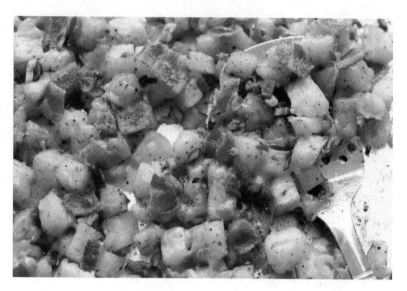

Ingredients for 4 people

- 12 new potatoes
- 12 slices of cooked smoked bacon
- Chilli powder

Preparation

1. Peel and wash the new potatoes. Boil them in a pot filled with lightly salted water or steam them.
2. Once the potatoes are cooked (you can check the cooking by inserting a toothpick: if the potato is soft it is ready) drain them and let them cool well.
3. Take the slices of bacon, preferably cut not too thin, and roll one around each potato. Place the potato and bacon bites on a baking sheet greased with oil or lined with baking paper and bake at 200 °C for 5-10 minutes.

4. Arrange three bites on each plate, sprinkle the surface with chili powder, without exaggerating, and top with a sauce to taste.

Spinach pie with spirulina cream

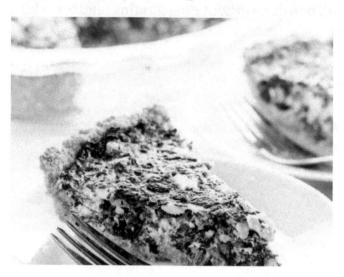

Ingredients for 4 people

For the flan

- 500 gr boiled and squeezed spinach
- 100 gr grated parmesan cheese
- 4 fresh eggs
- 1 tablespoon of olive oil
- Salt

For the cream:

- 100 gr grated parmesan cheese
- 250 gr milk
- 25 gr cornstarch or rice flour
- 25 gr butter
- 10 gr spirulina powder (gluten free)

Preparation

Flan preparation:

1. Blend the spinach, then in a bowl add it together with the other ingredients and with a whisk mix well until reduced to a creamy consistency.
2. Grease the moulds with butter and sprinkle with a little breadcrumbs (or rice flour, cornflour) to prevent the cakes from sticking during cooking.
3. Fill the molds with the mixture up to 2/3.
4. Bake in the oven at 180 degrees for about 30 minutes until risen and puffed up.

Preparation of the parmesan cream:

1. Heat the milk in a small saucepan until it comes to a boil, add the spirulina a little at a time, mixing well, after which turn off the flame.
2. In another saucepan melt the butter, add the flour and mix with a whisk until you obtain a smooth and homogeneous roux without lumps; add the milk continuing to mix with the whisk, over low heat.
3. Once the cream has thickened, remove from heat, add the grated Parmesan cheese and let it melt.
4. At this point, the pie can be served on a serving plate, pouring the cream over it and finishing with grated Parmesan cheese flakes.

Eggs with peas and bacon

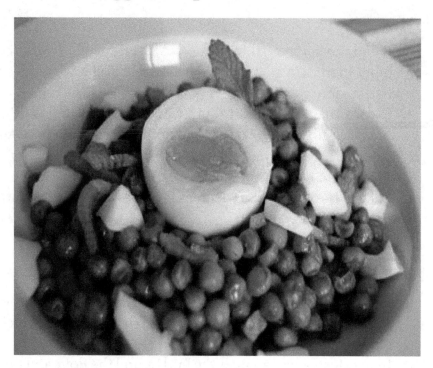

Ingredients for 4 people

- 800 grams of Peas
- 2 spring onions
- 300 grams of smoked bacon
- 4 Eggs
- 1 handful of Parsley
- Extra Virgin Olive Oil
- Salt
- Pepper
- Mint

Preparation

1. Clean the spring onions and slice them thinly, then sauté them in a non-stick pan with two tablespoons of oil. Add the diced bacon and brown it well.
2. Add the peas, season with salt and pepper, cover and cook for about 15-25 minutes, adding a few tablespoons of hot water if necessary. Meanwhile, finely chop the parsley and mint and add them a couple of minutes before the end of cooking, keeping a handful aside.
3. Place the eggs in a saucepan filled with water and boil for at least seven minutes from the time the water reaches a boil. Then place them under cold running water and peel them.
4. Distribute the peas and bacon on plates, cut the eggs in half and place two halves on each plate. Finish with a sprinkling of herbs and, if you like, a drizzle of extra virgin olive oil.

Asparagus and potato tortilla

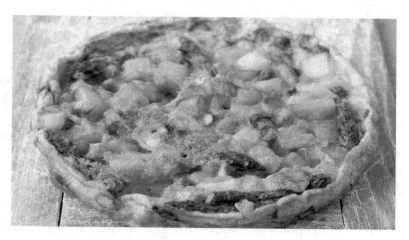

Ingredients for 4 people

- 500 grams of Asparagus
- 250 grams of Potatoes
- 150 grams of Onion
- 6 eggs
- 150 grams of Pasta Filata Cheese
- 1 bay leaf
- 50 grams of grated Grana Padano cheese
- Extra virgin olive oil
- Salt and Pepper

Preparation

1. Omelette ingredients should always be cooked and left to cool before adding the egg, otherwise the egg will cook but without giving the desired result, so start cooking the basic ingredients. Peel the potatoes and cut them into small cubes, then cook them in a pan with extra virgin olive oil

and bay leaf on high heat for about 7 minutes, until they become crispy on the outside but soft on the inside. As soon as they are ready, drain them and transfer them to a bowl where they will cool.

2. Peel the onions, slice them coarsely and cook them in a pan covered with a drizzle of oil for about 5 minutes being careful not to burn them, when they are cooked add them to the potatoes.

3. Finally, chop up the blanched asparagus and sauté them in a pan with a little oil, then add them to the potatoes and onions.

4. Once the ingredients are cold, beat the eggs and add them to the cooked vegetables with the Grana Padano, add salt and a pinch of pepper and mix everything together. Preheat the oven to 250 °C and begin assembling the tortilla: spread half of the mixture on a baking sheet about 20-22 cm in diameter, place the cheese slices on top and cover with the other half of the remaining mixture, then bake for about fifteen minutes, then take out of the oven and serve.

Bernese Sauce

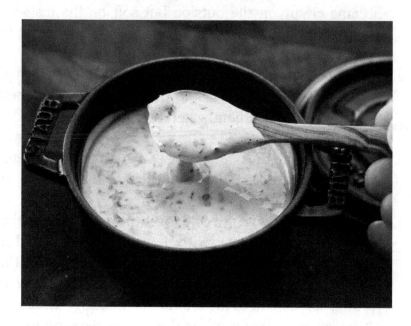

Ingredients for 4 people

- 3 Eggs
- 1 Shallot
- 200 grams of Butter
- 2 teaspoons of Tarragon
- 1 teaspoon of Pepper
- 60 millilitres of Vinegar
- Salt

Preparation

1. Finely chop the shallot and place in a small saucepan. Add the vinegar, half of the chopped tarragon, pepper and salt. Bring to a boil and cook over low heat until the mixture has reduced to one-third of its original amount.

2. Place a saucepan suitable for bain-marie cooking over a pot of water brought to a boil and kept on the stove over low heat. Strain the vinegar, shallot and tarragon mixture through a sieve, add the egg yolks and whisk together with a whisk until the mixture is smooth.

3. Add the chopped butter and continue to mix until the mixture has reached a creamy consistency.

4. Remove from the heat, pour the sauce into a glass bowl, season with salt, add the remaining tarragon and a pinch of pepper. Mix well and serve immediately.

Eggplant and bell pepper rolls

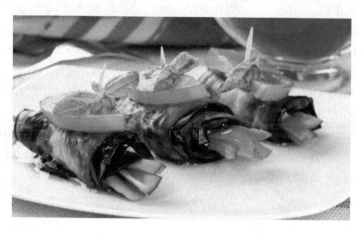

Ingredients for 4 people

- 2 Aubergines
- 2 Peppers
- 2 Tomatoes
- 1 handful of Basil
- Extra Virgin Olive Oil
- Salt

Preparation

6. In a bowl, pour three to four tablespoons of extra virgin olive oil, two pinches of salt and two to three coarsely chopped basil leaves. Mix everything together, cover with plastic wrap and let rest.
7. Thoroughly wash the eggplants, remove the two ends and cut them into slices about an inch thick lengthwise. Cook them on a hot cast iron griddle on both sides.

8. Wash the peppers, remove the stem and cut them in half. Remove the seeds and inner filaments, then cut them into strips.
9. With the help of a brush, preferably a silicone one, grease the eggplant with the basil-flavoured oil previously prepared. Take three to four strips of peppers, place them in the center of each slice of eggplant and roll them up.
10. Wash the tomatoes, cut them in half and then into slices and place one on top of each roulade, securing it with a toothpick. Top with fresh basil leaves.

Sweet potato and thyme quenelles

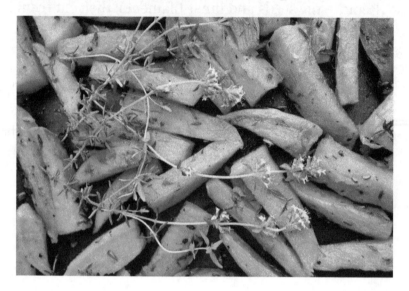

Ingredients for 4 people

- 1 kilo of sweet potatoes
- 20 grams of Maizena
- 1 handful of Thyme
- 1 Egg
- 3 tablespoons of Extra Virgin Olive Oil
- Salt

Preparation

4. Rinse and boil the sweet potatoes in plenty of cold salted water, along with a couple of sprigs of thyme. Once boiled and slightly cooled, peel and chop them, place them in a large bowl and mash them with a potato masher.

5. Add a few thyme leaves, the corn-starch, the oil, salt to taste and mix everything together. Finally add the egg and mix quickly.

6. Now create the quenelles with the help of two spoons of the same size and shape, better if wet, collect some of the dough with one of the two spoons and slide the dough on the other with a rotary movement of the spoons, trying to give the quenelles an elongated shape. Place them on a baking sheet with a drizzle of oil and bake for about 20 minutes at 190°-200°C.

Eggplants in oil

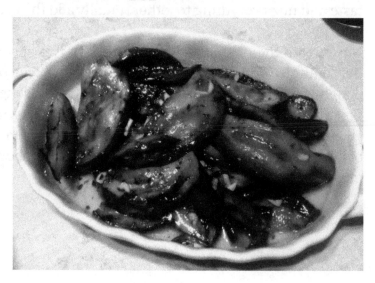

Ingredients for 8 people

- 2 kilos of eggplants
- 150 grams of fine salt
- 600 millilitres of white wine vinegar
- Seed Oil
- Oregano
- Fennel
- 6 cloves of Garlic

Preparation

1. Wash the eggplants well and remove the stalks, then peel them and cut them into strips about two inches long and one inch wide, about three millimetres thick. Place the eggplants in layers in a large, high-sided food container.

2. Sprinkle on each layer of eggplants a little bit of salt and, when you have finished arranging them, cover them with wine vinegar, then put a weight on top of the eggplants and leave them to rest covered by a cloth for three or four days. In this time the eggplants will undergo a sort of maceration with these two preservatives, that is salt and vinegar, and they will throw out all their vegetation water. After this time, the eggplants will be covered by a brine that you will drain off.

3. Squeeze out the remaining brine and place the eggplant in a bowl, then season with the fennel seeds and garlic, cleaned and finely chopped.

4. Continue seasoning with the oregano and stir until well combined. Pour the eggplant into the jar, leaving at least an inch and a half from the edge, and cover with oil. Wait a few minutes and you will notice that the eggplants will have occupied part of the space left free in the jar by absorbing part of the oil, then add more oil until well covered, after which close the jars and store them. The preserves will be good to eat after one week.

Gluten-free bread with rice flour

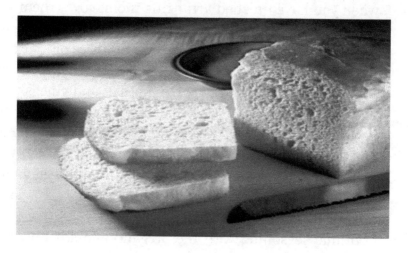

Ingredients for 4 people

- 350 millilitres of water
- 340 grams of rice flour
- 100 grams of potato starch
- 10 grams of dry brewer's yeast
- 2 tablespoons of Extra Virgin Olive Oil
- 1 teaspoon fine salt

Preparation

1. To make gluten-free bread with rice flour, place the water in the basket of the bread machine or planetary mixer, then add the salt and extra virgin olive oil.
2. Add the rice flour, potato starch and finally the dry brewer's yeast. Then knead for 20 minutes until the dough has reached the consistency of a loaf. Let it rise for 2 hours.
3. After the dough has risen, place the dough on a pastry board and shape the rolls, I had fun making them in the

shape of rice grains. Place the rolls on a baking sheet covered with parchment paper and let them rise for another 30 minutes.

4. After baking everything in a static oven at 180 degrees for 20 minutes, here is ready gluten-free bread with rice flour.

Caprese cake

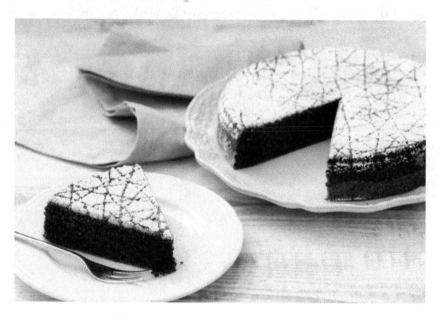

Ingredients for 6 people

- 400 grams of shelled Almonds
- 250 grams of Sugar
- 250 grams of Dark Chocolate
- 250 grams of Butter
- 6 Eggs
- 1 sachet of Vanillin
- Icing Sugar

Preparation

1. Cut the dark chocolate into small pieces and melt it in a bain-marie. With the help of a blender chop the almonds and mix them with the melted chocolate together with the vanillin.

2. Separate the yolks from the egg whites and cream the yolks with the sugar. Add the chocolate and almond mixture and mix well. Melt the butter and add it to the mixture.

3. Whip the egg whites until stiff and incorporate them into the mixture a little at a time, with the help of a spoon, with a movement from the bottom up so as not to disassemble the mixture.

4. Grease and flour a cake pan (ideally a round mold of about 30 cm) and pour the mixture inside. Bake in a preheated oven at 170 °C for about an hour. Once the cake is cooked, remove it from the oven, let it cool and dust the surface with powdered sugar.

APPENDIX

Cooking Conversion Charts

Volume (liquid)	
US Customary	Metric
1/8 teaspoon	0,6 ml
1/4 teaspoon	1.2 ml
1/2 teaspoon	2.5 ml
3/4 teaspoon	3.7 ml
1 teaspoon	5 ml
1 tablespoon	15 ml
2 tablespoon or 1 fluid ounce	30 ml
1/4 cup or 2 fluid ounces	59 ml
1/3 cup	79 ml
1/2 cup	118 ml
2/3 cup	158 ml
3/4 cup	177 ml
1 cup or 8 fluid ounces	237 ml
2 cups or 1 pint	473 ml
4 cups or 1 quart	946 ml
8 cups or 1/2 gallon	1.9 litres
1 gallon	3.8 litres

Weight (mass)	
US contemporary (ounces)	Metric (grams)
1/2 ounce	14 grams
1 ounce	28 grams
3 ounces	85 grams
3.53 ounces	100 grams
4 ounces	113 grams
8 ounces	227 grams
12 ounces	340 grams
16 ounces or 1 pound	454 grams

Oven Temperatures	
US contemporary	Metric
250° F	121° C
300° F	149° C
350° F	177° C
400° F	204° C
450° F	232° C

Volume Equivalents (liquid)		
3 teaspoons	1 tablespoon	0.5 fluid ounce
2 tablespoons	1/8 cup	1 fluid ounce
4 tablespoons	1/4 cup	2 fluid ounces
5 1/3 tablespoons	1/3 cup	2.7 fluid ounces
8 tablespoons	1/2 cup	4 fluid ounces
12 tablespoons	3/4 cup	6 fluid ounces
16 tablespoons	1 cup	8 fluid ounces
2 cups	1 pint	16 fluid ounces
2 pints	1 quart	32 fluid ounces
4 quarts	1 gallon	128 fluid ounces

CPSIA information can be obtained
at www.ICGtesting.com
Printed in the USA
LVHW021531110521
687091LV00003B/417

9 781802 534474